CW00701303

To all my patients who have taught me so much

To my friends and colleagues at Aetrex, especially Mr Peter Malkin and Mrs Whitney Alan
without whom this book would not have been possible

and

To Susan, Talita and Jemima for your constant inspiration, support and love

EASE THE FEET

Common foot disorders and how to address them

Dr George Ampat
Consultant Orthopaedic Surgeon

in association with
Aetrex, Inc.

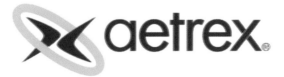

Contents

1. Introduction..5
2. Plantar Fasciitis 7
3. Metatarsalgia..9
4. Bunions...11
5. Diabetes and feet 14
6. Elderly & Foot Pain 19
7. Sports injuries 21
8. Arthritis...24
9. Should everyone wear orthotics? 27
10. Exercises for a healthy foot...33
11. References 45

DISCLAIMER

This book is intended to provide general educational information only. It is not meant to be used as a substitute for any type of professional medical advice. Each patient and condition are unique, and solutions, treatments, and results vary. Please do not rely on anything in this book without first seeking professional advice from a qualified physician or foot specialist.

Copyright © 2022 George Ampat
All rights reserved. No part of this publication may be reproduced, distributed, or transmitted in any form or by any means, including photocopying, recording or other electronic or mechanical methods without the prior written permission.

Talita Cumi Ltd
681, Liverpool Road, Southport PR8 3NS
www.ampat.co.uk   www.freefrompain.org.uk

Printed in the United Kingdon
Ampat, George
Ease The Feet
ISBN 978-0-9956769-6-1

Introduction

Why would I write a book on feet? Feet are a fundamental part of the human body. They support our whole body from the ground up and help us move around and participate in daily activities. Feet take us around the world and bring us home again. Without feet, we could not run to help others or walk arm in arm with our loved ones. And yet, 13 to 36% of us suffer from everyday foot pain [1].

Many people consider surgery a guaranteed solution to their pain. Unfortunately, the desired outcome is not always a reality. Surgery may actually cause further pain. Complications following foot and ankle surgery can be as high as 36% [2], with 10% of the patients being dissatisfied following surgery [3] and some 4.4 percent developing more severe and complex pain following surgery [4]. And, surgery cannot be undone. If you buy a house or a car that you do not like, you can sell it to off to someone else, maybe at a reduced price. But surgery is irreversible, and you cannot pass it on. Hence, we must explore all non-surgical options to treat foot pain before we consider surgery as an option.

Many non-surgical options are very effective. It's a matter of exploring your options and finding the right solution that works for you and your unique feet. In *Ease the Feet*, I outline common foot ailments, what causes each, and options for treatments. Orthotics are a simple and affordable solution to obtain relief without surgery. And

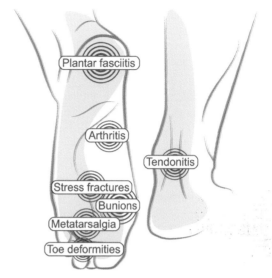

The various conditions that can contribute to foot pain

they work well for a variety of foot conditions and foot pain types.

In my own life, Aetrex Orthotics have been a life changer and maybe even a lifesaver. My family has a strong history of heart disease and heart attacks. Recent events put the fear of life into me. I wanted to become healthier by taking up cardiovascular activity. Unfortunately, I could not run because of gout. I had pain in my left foot and right knee. However, by using Aetrex Orthotics, I was able to start running. Slowly, I built up my fitness. I now weigh less, run regularly, and I'm much healthier overall. My running is slow, and I take about an hour to complete five kilometers.

But the difference is I *can* run. Aetrex Orthotics have given me that ability.

Many people like me have foot or musculoskeletal pain only when they are running. My advice to them is to use orthotics. It is like having a better tire when you are about to undertake a long car journey. Similarly, you need good support under your feet to run and stay healthy. The soft but firm orthotics from Aetrex creates natural conditions for the foot to keep your body aligned and supported. My own experience inspired me to write *Ease the Feet*. I want to help people with foot and ankle pain without resorting to surgical intervention, and I'm grateful for my partnership with Aetrex to bring this vital information to you.

In the different pages of this book various products from Aetrex are illustrated. These are provided as a guidance to enable you to choose an appropriate product. For detailed descriptions of individual products please use their web portal www.aetrex.com

DISCLAIMER

This book is intended to provide general educational information only. It is not meant to be used as a substitute for any type of professional medical advice. Each patient and condition are unique, and solutions, treatments, and results vary. Please do not rely on anything in this book without first seeking professional advice from a qualified physician or foot specialist.

DISCLOSURE

Please note that I have a commercial relationship with Aetrex. As part of that relationship I conduct research, write, speak at forums and run training sessions for Aetrex, Inc.

George Ampat, MBBS, MS & FRCS
Consultant Orthopaedic Surgeon
Liverpool, UK

1. Plantar Fasciitis

What is it?
Plantar fasciitis is the most common cause of heel pain. The plantar fascia is a piece of tissue connecting each of the toes with part of the heel bone. This tissue stabilises the arch of the foot and helps control movement. Plantar fasciitis occurs when this tissue is inflamed. Pain is usually felt in the heel and the arch of the foot in one or both feet. The pain is usually worst during the first steps of the day or following rest. Pain can also arise following walking, running, or standing for a long time.

Why does this occur?
Plantar fasciitis results from long-term pressure and repetitive strain on the foot from either

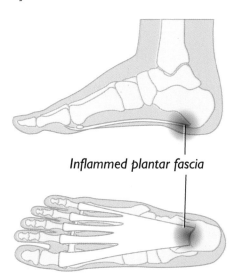

Inflammed plantar fascia

lifestyle, exercise, or old age. This repetitive strain leads to microtrauma, which leads to a repair response—the repetitive injury and repair cause chronic inflammation. There is often not a singular clear cause. People at greater risk of plantar fasciitis have tight calf muscles, high arched feet, or flat feet. It is also more common in overweight people and in people who frequently perform high-impact activities like running, dancing, or jumping.

How can it be treated?
Daily stretching of the plantar fascia and calf muscles can be helpful. Orthotics support the plantar fascia and decrease physical stress. Ice can be applied to the area of pain for 10-20 minutes at a time, up to three times per day. Steroid injections into the plantar fascia are also recommended, but unfortunately, steroid injections can damage the fat pad covering the heel. The fat pad then becomes thinner, and the condition can become more severe.

Orthotics?
Orthotics cradle the foot and decreases the repeated stress on the plantar fascia. This helps in reducing inflammation and the pain associated with plantar fasciitis.

Medication
If there is a definite trigger for the pain, like high-impact exercise, this can be decreased to reduce the pain. Over-the-counter anti-inflammatory medications like ibuprofen may provide some relief in the short term.

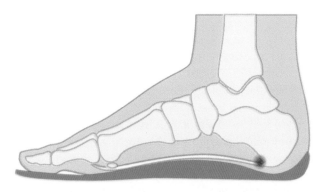

Contoured Orthotics cradle the foot and decrease the repetitive stress on the Plantar fascia. This combined with stretching results in 90% of patients obtaining relief.

Surgery

With non-operative treatment, 90% of patients will have relief of symptoms within 12 months. If there is no relief with the above methods, surgery can be considered. Recently more success has been achieved by releasing the inner calf muscle rather than the plantar fascia.

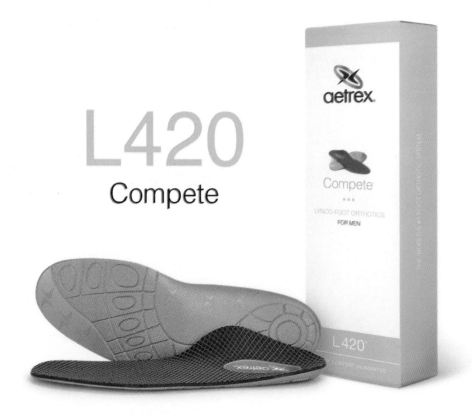

L420
Compete

2. Metatarsalgia

What is it?

Metatarsalgia is defined as pain in the ball of the foot (the front of the foot where the toes meet the feet) directly beneath the metatarsal heads. The metatarsal heads are the joints that connect the foot to the toes. They support weight and, as such, they can be a target for pain and inflammation due to the pressure they are often under when we walk, run and stand. Estimates of the prevalence of foot pain in the metatarsal region range from 5% to 36%. The severity of the condition is affected by the variation in pressure applied to the forefoot. These differences in pressure are increased by factors including the shape of the feet (length of the metatarsals and high arch), tightness of the calf muscles, unsupportive footwear, taking part in excessive physical exercise and age.

Why does this occur?

Based on how it is caused, there are three types of metatarsalgia - primary, secondary, and iatrogenic. Primary metatarsalgia is due to anatomical variations. The 1st metatarsal may be shorter and allow greater forces to be transferred via the 2nd, 3rd, and 4th metatarsals. The 2nd, 3rd, and 4th metatarsals are thinner and cannot take the excessive strain, resulting in pain. Tightness of the calf muscles (the gastrocnemius) and a high arch can also cause primary metatarsalgia. Secondary metatarsalgia is caused by conditions that increase the pressure on the metatarsal joints indirectly. This occurs in conditions like Rheumatoid Arthritis (RA), where the plantar pad (the thick flesh under the heads of the metatarsal) moves away, reducing the amount of soft tissue cushioning the bones. Due to the decrease in the amount of soft tissue covering the heads of the metatarsals, it becomes painful when one bears weight. The third category is called iatrogenic, which means it has been caused by previous medical intervention.

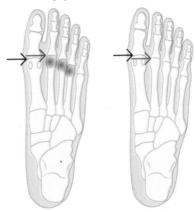

The image on the left shows that the 2nd , 3rd and 4th metatarsals (red arrow) are longer than the 1st (black arrow). The image on the right shows normal lengths of the metatarsals.

For example, surgery to correct bunions may shorten the first metatarsal causing increased weight and pressure on the other metatarsals.

In addition, there is another cause of metatarsalgia, Morton's neuroma. Due to repeated compression from wearing a tight shoe, a nerve in the foot becomes swollen and inflamed. This usually affects the area between the 3rd and 4th toes.

9

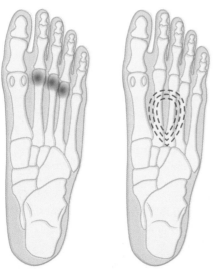

The metatarsal pad takes away the pressure from the heads of the metatarsals and provides relief

How can it be treated?
Stretching
Stretches that increase the flexibility of the calf muscles (gastrocnemius) are recommended.

Orthotics
Metatarsal pads, which provide support behind the ball of the foot, have been found to relieve the pressure on the metatarsals by up to 60%.

Surgery
In severe cases, surgery may be required. Various surgical procedures have been described, including the release of the tight calf muscle, shortening of the 2nd, 3rd and 4th metatarsals, excision of the neuroma etc.

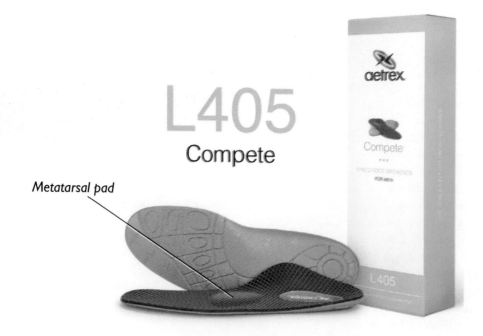

Metatarsal pad

3. Bunions

What is it?

A bunion is a deformity of the joint at the base of the big toe. Medically this is known as Hallux Valgus. One in three to five individuals develop this deformity. The condition is 15 times more frequent in women and is the most common deformity in the ball of the foot. There are two components to the deformity. Initially, the metatarsal starts to point inwards, with which the great toe begins to point outwards. This results in the metatarsal head becoming protuberant and inflamed. When the bunion becomes more prominent, the body creates a small fluid-filled sack called a bursa over the deformity to act as a cushion. The deformity itself does not cause discomfort, but the bursa becomes inflamed, causing pain. The collapse of the arch is associated with bunion formation.

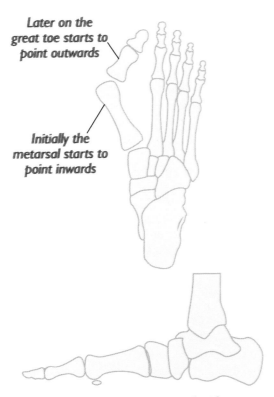

Later on the great toe starts to point outwards

Initially the metarsal starts to point inwards

The bunion is associated with collapse of the arch

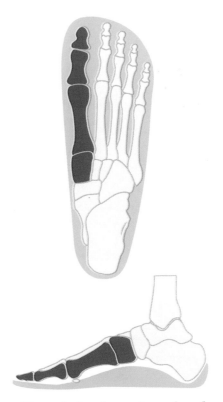

The orthotics elevate the arch and help to realign the bones

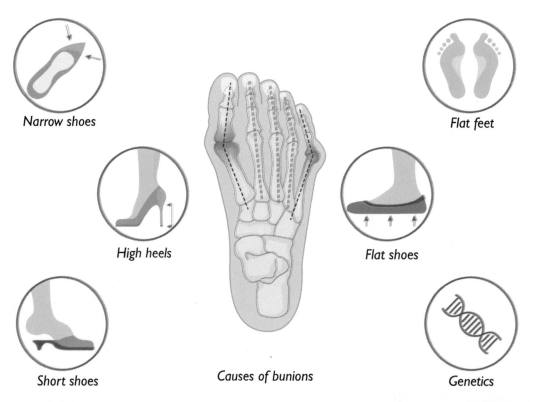

Narrow shoes

Flat feet

High heels

Flat shoes

Short shoes

Causes of bunions

Genetics

Why does this occur?

The causes of the condition are not completely clear. There seems to be an evolutionary basis for the condition. Humans descended from apes. In apes, this deformity is natural and allows them to hold onto branches and climb trees. When humans evolved from apes, the great toe straightened out as an adaptation for walking and running on the ground. The deformity that occurs in bunions is similar to the natural structure seen in apes. In addition, genetics also play a role, and this condition runs in families. There are other risk factors like wearing narrow shoes and high-heels and footwear with pointed toe boxes. It is likely that individuals with a genetic predisposition who also have the risk factors are even more likely to develop this deformity. Age is an additional risk factor, and seniors have a greater incidence of bunions. As one ages, the ligaments and other soft tissues weaken, and the arch collapses. As the arch collapses, the bunion becomes apparent.

How can it be treated?

Painful bunions can be treated by wearing proper shoes which provides space for the deformity. Footwear that accommodates the deformity will reduce the pressure on the bursa and decrease inflammation and pain.

Orthotics

Orthotics support the arch and prevent the metatarsal from deviating inwards. This, in turn, will prevent the great toe from deviating outwards. In addition the arch support decreases the pressure and pain at the bunion by redirecting and redistributing the pressure to other areas of the foot.

Surgery

If a permanent deformity has to be corrected, surgery may be required. Many forms and combinations of surgery can be carried out depending on the severity of the condition.

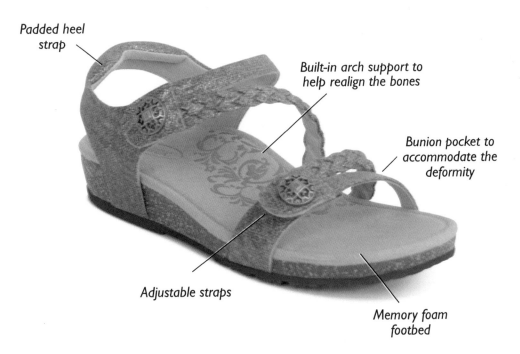

Padded heel strap

Built-in arch support to help realign the bones

Bunion pocket to accommodate the deformity

Adjustable straps

Memory foam footbed

The Aetrex Jillian has a lot of features that help with bunion deformity

4. Diabetes and feet

What is it?

Diabetes occurs when the body is not able to control glucose levels. Our bodies are made up of billions of cells. The cells require fuel or energy. Glucose is one of the fuels used by the body. Insulin is needed to move the glucose from outside the cell to inside the cell. This is similar to the pump in a fuel forecourt. Though there is fuel in the fuel forecourt, a pump is needed to pump it into the car. In diabetes, there is a lot of glucose in the blood due to a lack of insulin or an inability of the insulin to transport the glucose into the cell.

There are two types of diabetes. Type 1 diabetes is an autoimmune disease where the body's immune system destroys the insulin-producing pancreatic beta cells. Type 2 diabetes occurs when insulin becomes ineffective or inadequate. Lifestyle conditions like obesity and inactivity cause Type 2 diabetes. High blood sugar levels can result in damage to the nerves, kidneys, and eyes. The heart can also be affected, and people with diabetes have an increased risk of angina and heart attacks. The incidence of diabetes is increasing worldwide. According to estimates from 2019, 463 million people worldwide were reported to be living with this condition.

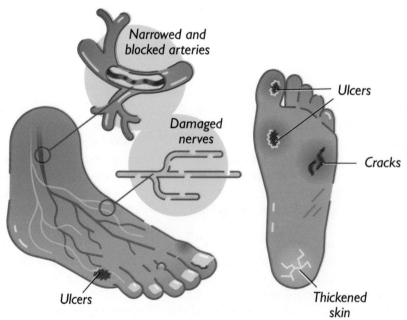

Narrowed and blocked arteries

Damaged nerves

Ulcers

Cracks

Ulcers

Thickened skin

Damage caused by diabetes to the feet

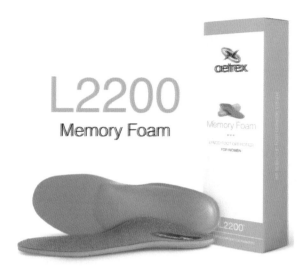

L2200
Memory Foam

Memory foam Orthotics for superior cushioning. Arch support helps to redistribute the weight and ease stress at pressure points.

Unfortunately, diabetes affects the feet and can cause serious problems. Initially, the small nerves in the feet are affected, causing numbness or a lack of sensation. The lack of sensation allows damage to the skin to go unnoticed. In addition, there is a decreased ability to heal, which allows the damage to become an ulcer. An ulcer may initially only be on the surface, but it can become deep and involve the tendons and bones. A very deep ulcer with infection in the bone may require amputation. The statistics are quite grim. 1 in 6 diabetics will develop an ulcer. 1 in 6 who have an ulcer will ultimately undergo a leg amputation. 50% of the patients with an amputation will die within five years.

How can it be treated?
The main issue is to treat the diabetes and keep blood sugar levels under control. The second issue is to avoid developing an ulcer.

Orthotics
Normally when standing on a flat surface like the inside of a shoe, most of the weight-bearing occurs only through the ball of the feet and the heel. Orthotics contoured to the feet allow the body weight to be distributed over a wider surface area and not just through the heel and the ball of the foot. This relieves the pressure on the parts of the foot which are more prone to ulcerations. Research has shown that orthotics reduce both the occurrence and the recurrence of ulcers. Orthotics have also been found to reduce the threat of amputation from 54% to 6%. However, once an ulcer develops, specialist treatment is required.

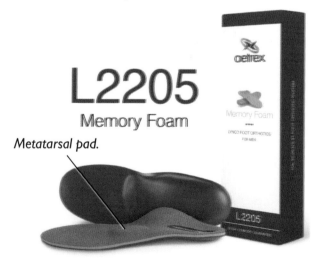

L2205
Memory Foam

Metatarsal pad.

Memory foam Orthotics with metatarsal pads allowing for additional pressure relief in the front of the foot.

Important
Inspect the sole of the foot regularly

Individuals with diabetes should inspect the sole of the feet regularly. To see the sole of the feet is difficult. Leaning a mirror onto the side of a wall will allow inspection of the sole of the feet for any cracks, thickening of the skin or ulcers. If any abnormality is noticed, it is best to seek professional medical advice. Please ensure to place the mirror securely and take extra care to prevent any injury. Mirrors are heavy and are sharp if they break. Keeping the mirrors on floor level increases the chance of breakage and injury. Hence extra caution is required.

Ask a friend / relative to test the feeling in the toes regularly.

Testing the sensation in the toes is important to find out if there is neuropathy. Neuropathy occurs when diabetes damages the nerves and parts of the foot become numb. The toes are the first place to develop numbness as they are farthest from the brain. Numbness is harmful because pain is protective. Pain prevents us from damaging parts of the body. If pain sensation is lost, then injury or damage is not recognised and deep infection can occur.

A friend or a relative can help to test if there is numbness / neuropathy in the toes. Look away and ask the friend or relative to lightly touch each of the toes. The touch should be light with the finger tip and should not cause the toes to move. Normally the light touch can be felt. If the touch is not felt then neuropathy might have occurred and it is important to seek professional medical advice.

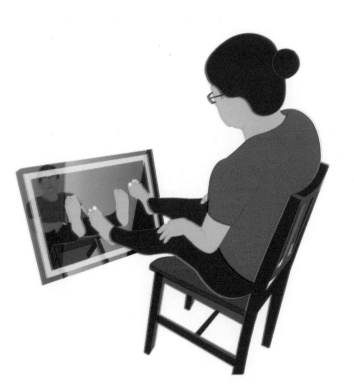

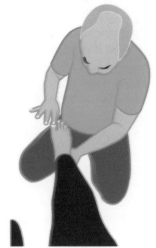

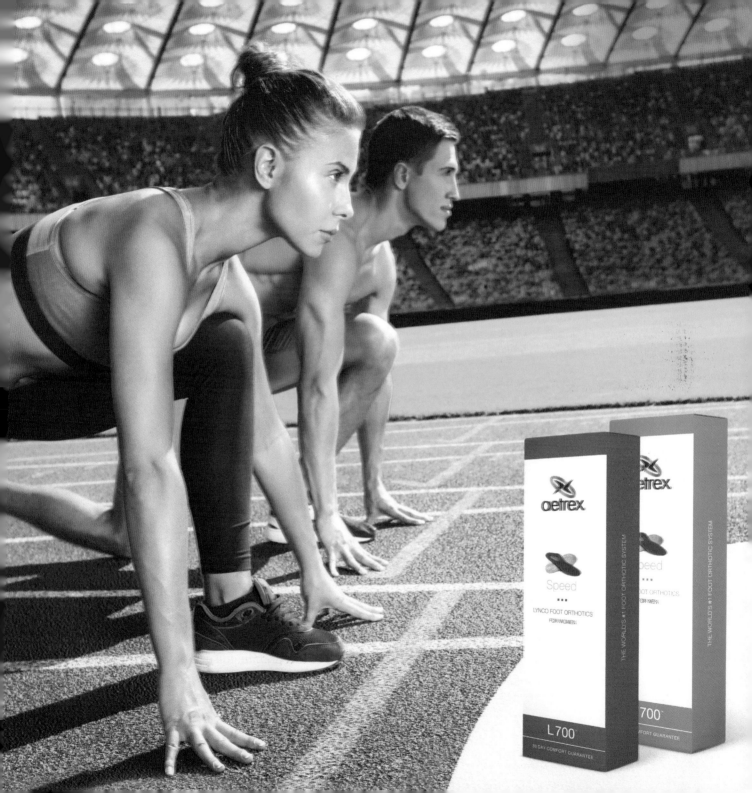

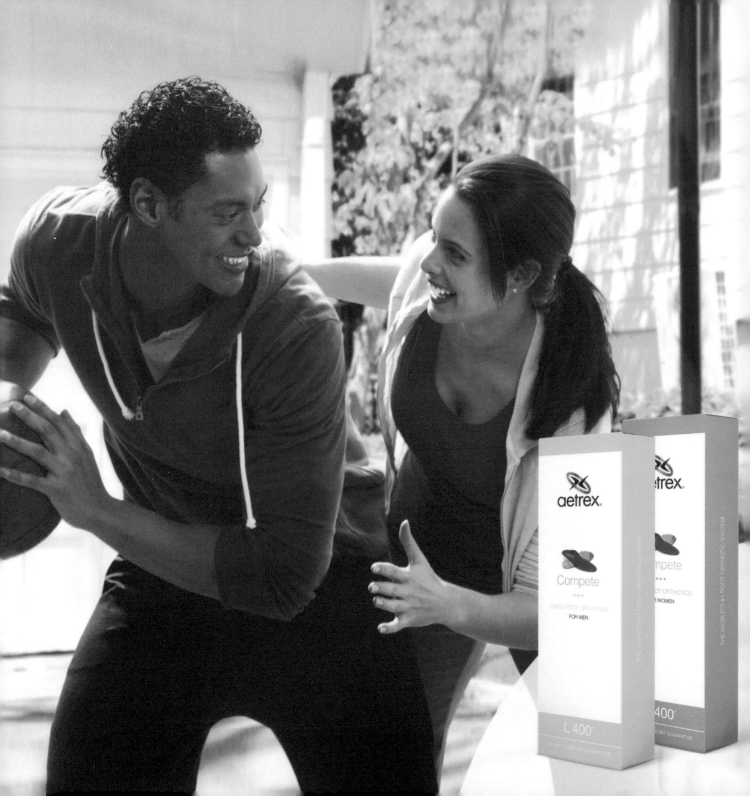

5. Elderly & Foot Pain

What is it?
The foot is subjected to extreme amounts of repetitive pressure and stress every day. It is therefore not surprising that pain in the feet is a common problem, especially in older populations. It has been estimated that 24% of people over the age of 45 will have foot pain, with symptoms more frequent in women than men. Foot pain in seniors is associated with decreased walking, decreased mobility and thereby a decrease in independence. 20% of older people with foot pain blame their symptoms as the main reason they cannot leave the house. A decrease in the ability to balance is also an issue in seniors.

Why does this occur?
With ageing, the muscles and tendons slowly weaken and do not support the foot. These conditions can indirectly cause corns,

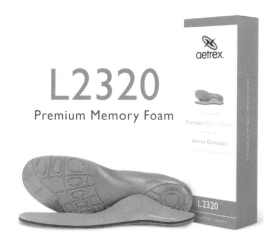

Premium L2320 has extra cushioning on the inner side of the heel to help with conditions like plantar fasciitis

calluses, bunions, hammer toes and claw toes. Obesity and female gender are also risk factors for foot pain. A vicious cycle sets in as one ages. Pain decreases mobility; decreased mobility leads to weakness of the muscles; weakness in the muscles leads to a decrease in balance; a decrease in balance leads to increased falls and injuries; and falls and injuries increase pain.

How can it be treated?
Change in footwear
We all like to buy shoes that are "eye-friendly" and not "feet-friendly". As a result, 95% of footwear primarily serves the eye and not the feet. Only 5% of everyday footwear are designed to serve the feet primarily. Given the association between footwear choice and foot pain, the most effective intervention is the most simple –

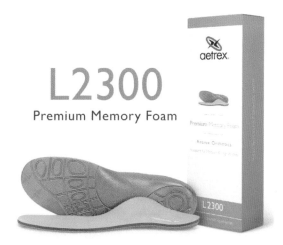

Premimum memory foam Orthotics help provide support and pain relief

changing footwear. One study investigated the effects of footwear on disabling foot pain of community-dwelling older people. The intervention group received off-the-shelf, extra-depth footwear with a compliant upper, whilst the control group received usual care. The study found that, after four months, the intervention group had a more significant reduction in foot pain and developed fewer foot lesions than the control group.

the pressure on painful regions of the foot. Orthotics with heel cups can decrease heel pain. Orthotics with metatarsal pads can reduce pain in the front of the foot. Orthotics may also decrease pressure on the toes. Balance is dependent on the brain receiving sensory input from the eyes, the semi circular canals in the inner ears and from the peripheral sensory receptors in the feet and legs. We commonly recognise five senses. They are vision, hearing, taste, smell, and touch. Balance relies on another sensation called proprioception. Proprioception is joint position sense. As one foot lands while walking, that foot sends impulses to the brain about the ground. That sensory input allows the brain to position the next foot. Wearing orthotics increases the surface area of the foot that is in contact with the ground and increases this sensory input. The increased sensory input helps the brain to steady the body and thereby decreases the incidence of falls.

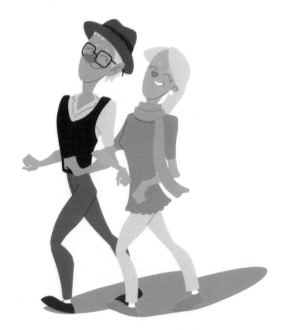

Wearing Orthotics decreases pain and improves balance. The pain relief enables frequent walks and increased physical activity to improve cardiovascular fitness.

Orthotics
Orthotics allow the body weight to be distributed over a wider area, thereby decreasing

6. Sports injuries

Medial tibial stress syndrome, stress fractures and Patellofemoral pain syndrome

What is it?
Medial tibial stress syndrome causes pain in the lower part of the leg along the inner border of the larger bone (tibia).

Stress fractures are minor fractures that occur within the substance of the bone. This occurs mainly in the lower part of the shinbone (tibia), metatarsals, navicular, fibula, and femur.

Patellofemoral pain syndrome is pain that occurs around the knee and is more frequently seen in female athletes and runners.

Why does this occur?
Medial tibial stress syndrome is caused by the repeated activity of the lower leg muscles that arise from the back of the main lower leg bone (Tibia). These muscles help with walking, running and maintenance of the arch. Excessive and repetitive use of these muscles pulls the fibres of these muscles at their attachment to the bone.

Stress fractures occur when the body is not able to keep up with the repetitive damage and repair of numerous minor fractures. Bone consists of flexible collagen fibres that are hardened with calcium. This is similar to reinforced concrete which has steel cables and cement. The collagen takes the place of the steel cables, and the calcium takes the place of the cement. If a bone is subjected to a very large load like a 100 kg weight falling onto it, it will likely break completely. That would be a fracture. However, if the bone is subjected to repetitive small loads, only a few fibres may break. The body immediately tries to heal up the few fibres that have broken. Unfortunately, at times the repetitive stress may break more fibres than what the body can repair. This is a stress fracture.

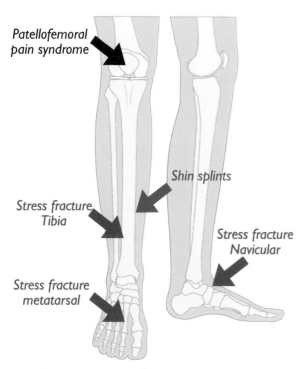

Patellofemoral pain syndrome

Shin splints

Stress fracture Tibia

Stress fracture Navicular

Stress fracture metatarsal

Common sites of sports injuries

Patellofemoral pain syndrome occurs when the kneecap repeatedly rubs against the lower end of the femur. Together, the femur, the tibia and the kneecap form the knee joint. Many factors may cause patellofemoral pain syndrome, but pronation of the foot is mainly implicated. Pronation of the foot causes internal rotation of the tibia and internal rotation of the femur. This occurs because all these bones are attached to one another and form a part of the same chain. The forces on one are transferred to the others like falling dominoes. But as the femur and tibia roll inwards, the quadriceps muscle in front of the thigh pulls the kneecap outwards. The repetitive friction as   kneecap is pulled outwards while the knee joint rolls inwards causes patellofemoral pain syndrome.

How can it be treated?

Severe pain from any of the above conditions requires reducing or even stopping the repetitive activity, pain killers, ice, therapy, and splints. Once healed, there can be a slow return to activity.

Stretching and strengthening exercises may be required. Treatment from a qualified health professional is recommended as there may be other underlying issues.

The clever plan would be to avoid these conditions. Wearing orthotics decreases pronation and the collapse of the arch. Decreasing the collapse of the arch reduces the load on the muscle pulling up the arch,

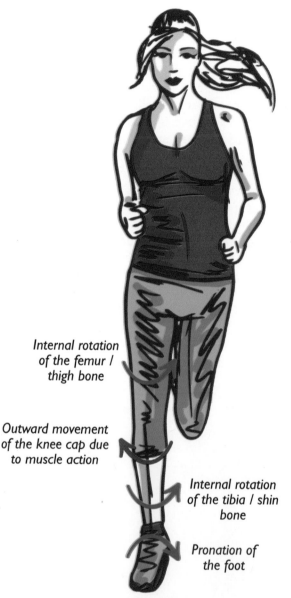

Internal rotation of the femur / thigh bone

Outward movement of the knee cap due to muscle action

Internal rotation of the tibia / shin bone

Pronation of the foot

Domino effect when running. What happens in the foot gets transmitted upwards

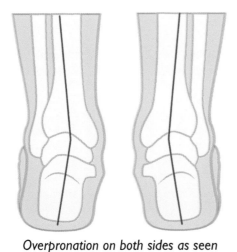

Overpronation on both sides as seen from behind

Overpronation corrected with appropriate Orthotics

thereby preventing or decreasing the chance of developing medial tibial stress syndrome.

Similarly, preventing pronation decreases the inward rotation of the tibia and the femur, which will reduce the repetitive stress between the kneecap and the lower end of the femur. This will help to prevent patellofemoral syndrome.

In addition, orthotics cradle the foot and allow for shock absorption, which decreases the chances of developing stress fractures.

7. Arthritis

What is it?

Arthritis is inflammation of the joint(s). The inflammation causes pain and discomfort, which can reduce mobility. The cartilage is the smooth, shiny surface at the ends of the bones. In advanced cases of arthritis, the inflammation may result in the complete damage of the affected joints with a total loss of cartilage. This can then result in raw bone rubbing against raw bone.

Why does this occur?

Arthritis may occur for two reasons. Firstly, it can be from wear and tear and is then called osteoarthritis. The other is inflammatory arthritis, where the body's immune mechanism needlessly attacks the joint. The most common inflammatory arthritis that affects the feet is Rheumatoid arthritis. Sometimes inflammation may also result from excess deposition of uric acid in the joints following gout. There are four sites which are usually affected by arthritis in the feet. The most common is the ankle joint, and this is mainly after injury. The mild misalignment from the injury causes excessive wear of the cartilage and results in osteoarthritis. The second is in the ball of the foot at the base of the great toe. This is usually the result of gout. The third is below the ankle in the subtalar joint, and that is mainly caused by the collapse of the arch as one ages. The fourth area is the middle of the foot and may also occur following injury.

How can it be treated?
Lifestyle changes

Gout can be helped by adopting a healthier lifestyle. Drinking more water, eating fewer rich foods, and exercising more can help reduce symptoms.

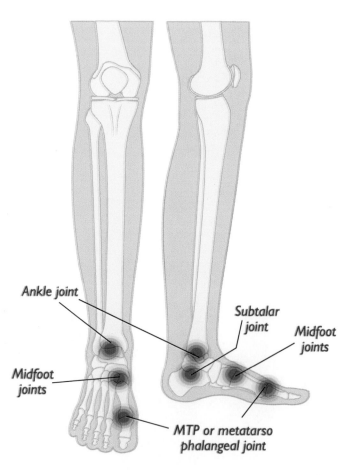

Sites of arthritis in the foot
and ankle

L2400
Customizable

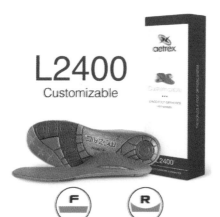

Forefoot - Neutal
Rearfoot - Cupped
Standard orthotic for everyday use or mid foot pain

L2405
Customizable

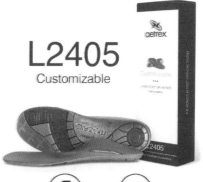

Forefoot - Metatarsal pad
Rearfoot - Cupped
For pain in the forefoot - metarsalgia

L2420
Customizable

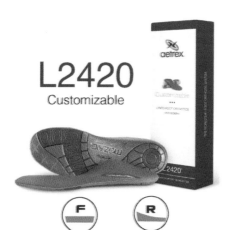

Forefoot - Neutal
Rearfoot - Posted
For flexible flatfeet or rearfoot pain

L2425
Customizable

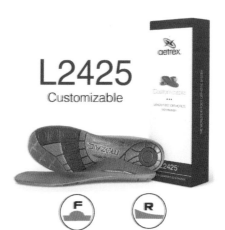

Forefoot - Metatarsal pad
Rearfoot - Posted
For pain both in the rearfoot and forefoot

Each style of Aetrex Orthotics come in 4 different configurations. The four different configurations are a combination of 2 forefoot options (Neutral / Metatarsal pad) and 2 rear foot options (Cupped and Posted). The posted Orthotic is built up on the inner side at the heel.

Orthotics?

Pain in the front of the feet can be helped by using orthotics with a metatarsal pad. Arthritis in the middle and the back of the foot can be helped by using an orthotic with an arch support.

Footwear modification

Stiffening the front part of the shoe helps to restrict movement in the ball of the foot. Using a slightly boat-shaped shoe decreases movement in the arthritic joint as the shape of the shoe allows it to absorb some of the rocking motion that is required during normal walking.

Surgery

In advanced cases, surgery may be required. Injections of steroids and local anaesthetic not only decrease pain but also help identify and confirm the joints involved. If the injection does not relieve the pain, even for a short time, then the area injected is not where the pain is arising from. This information can guide surgical intervention. There are four surgical options. 1. Debridement – trimming of the excess bone that forms around the joint, 2. Osteotomy – Cutting the bone and realigning them in a better position, 3. Fusion – removing the cartilage and making two bones into one using screws and or plates, and 4. Replacement – changing the joint with an artificial joint. Success rates can vary, and all surgical procedures can result in failure and complications.

8. Should everyone wear orthotics?

Twenty-four percent (24%) of the population have foot and/or ankle pain. That makes it 1 in 4 adults. Let us look at why foot pain is a common problem. Let us look at the past, many thousands of years ago, a time when we did not have shoes and walked barefoot. A time when we did not have roads, cities or hard-floored buildings. A time when we walked on soft surfaces such as grass, soil, and sand. Our foot was designed by nature to walk on soft ground. When walking on soft ground, the earth moulds to the shape of the foot.

Imagine walking on a sandy beach and creating footprints on the sand. As gravity pulls us toward

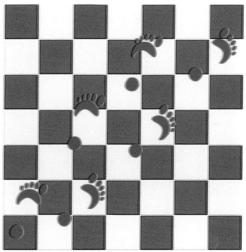

Footprints on a hard surface are small. The decreased area increases the pressure.

Footprints on a sandy beach are large. The increased area decreases the pressure.

the ground, the pressure of our weight is evenly distributed across the plane of our feet, and there is a wide area of contact. This is not the case when we walk on hard surfaces such as a tiled floor. On a tiled floor or on a hard surface, the contact area between the feet and the ground is less. A similar situation occurs when we wear shoes. This is because the inside of the shoe is also flat and is not contoured like an orthotic.

What can walking on flat and hard surfaces do to our feet?
Our feet are flexible and tend to turn inwards when we walk or stand. This movement when our feet turn in is called overpronation. Overpronation causes the arches to flatten and the ankles to collapse inwards. Most of us can cope with walking on flat surfaces as our muscles

and ligaments are strong. But 1 in 4 cannot and will have pain. Problems with incorrect foot position can also have a domino effect on the ankles, knees, hips, and even the back, resulting in pain or discomfort in areas distant to the feet.

How can orthotics help?
Orthotics lift the arch, cushion the sole, and evenly redistribute the pressure under the feet. Science tells us that pressure is force divided by area, i.e. Pressure = Force / Area. This means that if we increase the area that our foot comes into contact with, the pressure (and therefore the pain) can be reduced.

When we walk on hard surfaces like a tiled floor,

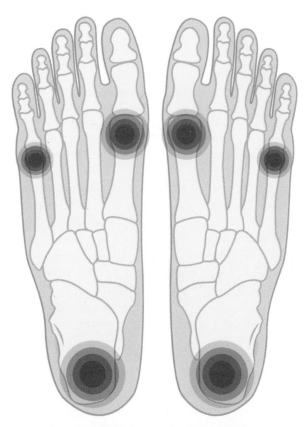

Increased pressure and greater weight transmission at three points when walking on a flat hard surface

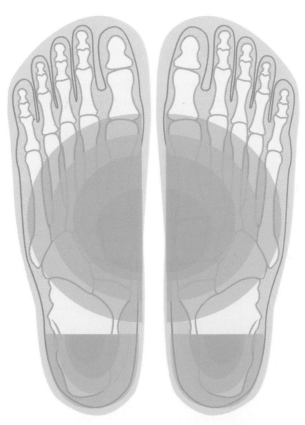

Pressure is equally distributed when walking on a contoured surface. Similar to using soft and firm orthotics with arch support and a cupped heel

the contact area is less. The smaller area of contact increases the pressure through the parts of the foot that are in contact with the floor as the weight of our body remains the same. However, as we walk on soft ground, the ground gives way slightly, and there is a greater contact area. The ground giving way and moulding to the shape of our feet is clearly seen when we walk on a sandy beach. The majority of foot pain can be managed effectively by providing the feet with a proper contoured surface to rest on. This is how orthotics provide our feet with a comfortable platform to walk and run on.

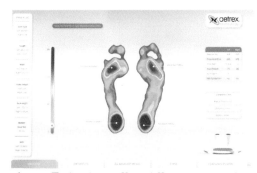

Aetrex Technology offers different types of scanners. Some provide a static reading of the pressure the feet apply to the ground. Some analyse one's pressure when walking. Others measure various 3D measurements of the feet, not just the force transmitted to the floor.

$$\textbf{Pressure} = \frac{\textbf{Force}}{\textbf{Area}}$$

With orthotics, you can wear your favourite shoe.

Studies have shown that one of the factors that deter individuals from orthopaedic shoes is the 'attractiveness' of the footwear. However, orthotics can be placed inside your shoe and allow you to wear your favourite footwear and feel great while you do it! However, your footwear may need to be slightly roomier to accommodate the orthotics.

Is scanning your foot important?

A good way to see how foot scanning can help with pain is to compare this to fitting tires in the car. When tires are fitted, they are balanced and aligned. Balancing and aligning the tire makes the tire last longer. The vehicle also becomes more fuel-efficient. Tires are expensive to replace, so we are diligent in balancing and aligning them. However, it seems that since our feet are part of our bodies and not something we paid for, we are not so diligent in balancing and aligning them. If balancing and aligning car tires improve efficiency and decrease wear of the tire, it then stands to reason that balancing and aligning the feet may produce similar results. The art of scanning the feet is called pedobarography.

Do our feet or our car tires travel a greater distance in their lifetime?

An average car tire travels 20,000 miles. Our feet on the other hand, cover approximately 110,000 miles in a lifetime, which is the equivalent of travelling four times around the globe! It is easy to neglect our feet which can cause problems and ultimately foot pain down the line. Scanning the feet can identify the type of orthotic required.

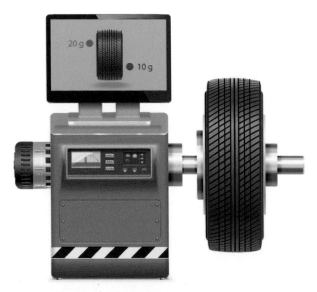

If our tires require balancing, our feet require scanning to understand how to better offload pressure. Our feet are more valuable than car tires.

The correct orthotics will cradle our foot and provide the support and comfort our feet require to stay healthy. Aetrex Technology offers a variety of 3D and pressure-based foot scanners that provide a pedobarograph. These foot scanners can identify arch types and define high-pressure points. Following the foot scan, the software provides an image showing the pressure reading across both the feet.

Aetrex scanners also provide orthotic suggestions best suited for each foot type based on one's individual scan.

Summary

If we take great care and invest in having high-quality tires for our car, then it stands to reason that we need a high-quality surface for our feet to walk on. We have no control of the outside environment. However, we do have control of the inside of our shoes. If using an orthotic is like walking on a sandy beach, then it is essential that we have that contoured surface inside our shoes. Wearing an orthotic is like creating nature inside our shoes. It is like taking a slice of sand from the beach and inserting it into our shoes to walk everywhere. Having a high-quality surface for our feet to tread by using orthotics will give us more pain-free mileage from our feet. This is the reason why I recommend foot orthotics for everyone.

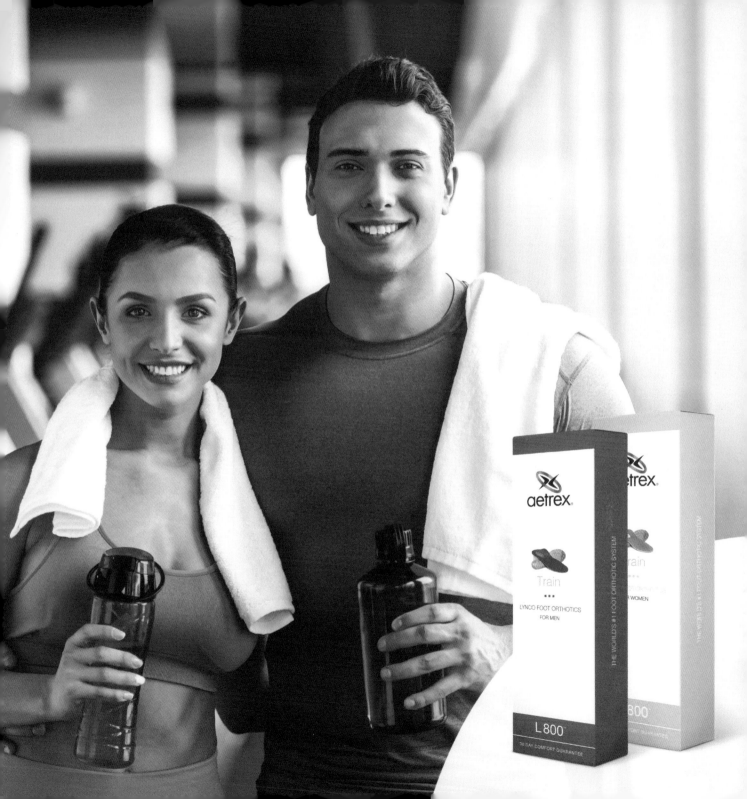

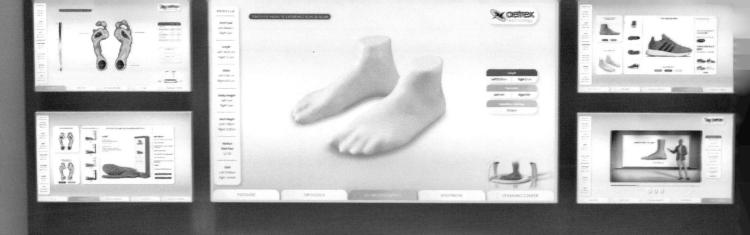
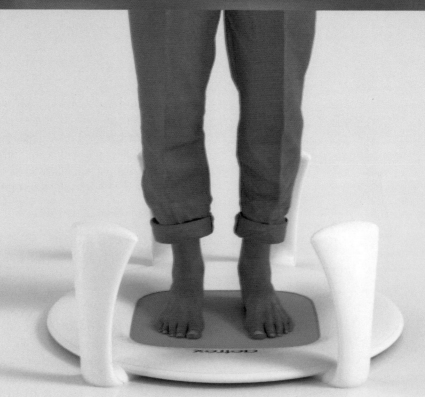

Exercises for a healthy foot

Either all the exercises or a combination of them can be performed. Please do not do the exercise if it is causing pain. Some discomfort can be expected when exercising but DO NOT do the exercise if it is causing pain. Discomfort is acceptable but pain is not acceptable. Only slowly and gradually, over a period of time, should one increase the intensity and repetition of the exercises.

Stretching exercises

---

1. Plantar Fascia Stretch

Begin by sitting on a chair. Cross one leg over the other. Grab the base of the toes of the crossed leg with one hand and pull the toes back toward the shin until a stretch is felt in the arch or plantar fascia. Push on the arch at the heel with the thumb of the other hand. The thumb should be able to feel the tension in the plantar fascia. Hold the stretch for a count of 10. Repeat x 3. Repeat x 3 on the other leg.

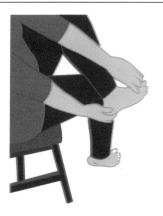

---

2. Inversion

Sit on a chair with feet flat on the floor. Now roll the feet inwards by lifting the inside of the feet. Attempt to face the soles with each other. Maintain this position for a count of 10. Then lower the inside of the feet until they are flat on the floor. Repeat x 3.

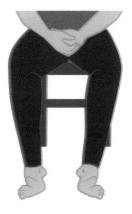

---

3. Eversion

Sit on a chair with feet flat on the floor. Now roll the feet outwards by lifting the outside of the feet. Attempt to face the soles away from each other. Maintain this position for a count of 10. Then lower the outside of the feet until they are flat on the floor. Repeat x 3.

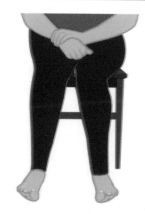

4. Wall Stretch

Stand facing a wall, about one and a half foot lengths away. With outstretched arms, place both hands on the wall at shoulder height. Lean forward so that the chest and then the hips touch the wall. Keep the heels planted on the floor while leaning forward. Feel the stretch down the back of the legs. Hold for a count of 10. Repeat x 3.

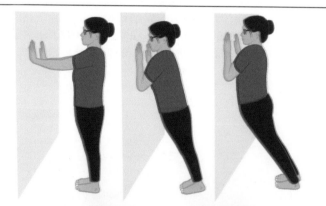

5. Step Stretch

Stand on a step with only the toes and balls (front of the feet) placed on the step. Hold the bannister for support. Now slowly allow the heels to drop below the level of the step. Feel the stretch down the back of the calves. Maintain the lowered stretched position for a count of 10. Return to normal. Repeat x 3.

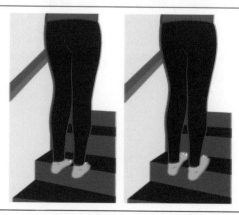

6. Calf Stretch:

Perch on the edge of a chair. Straighten one leg until the knee is straight and the heel is on the floor. The other foot should remain flat on the floor to provide stability. Now, pull the foot of the straight leg towards the shin as much as possible. Feel the stretch in the back of the calf. Hold for a count of 10. Repeat x 3. Repeat x 3 on the other leg.

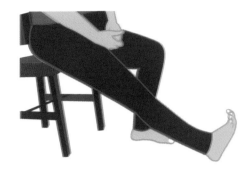

7. Hamstring Stretch:

Perch on the edge of a chair. Straighten one leg until the knee is straight and the heel is on the floor. The other foot should remain flat on the floor to provide stability. Place both hands on the thigh of the straight leg. Keep the back as straight as possible, and slowly slide the hands down the straight leg as much as possible. Feel the stretch in the back of the thigh. Hold for a count of 10. Repeat x 3. Repeat x 3 on the other leg.

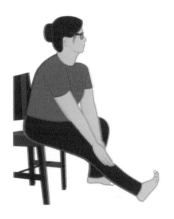

8. Foot Roll Out

Stand beside a sofa. Hold the arm of the sofa / couch to maintain balance. Raise the foot closest to the couch off the ground and stand only on the opposite leg. Place the outer aspect of the raised foot against the side of the sofa / couch. Now push the foot outwards and into the couch. Hold this position for a count of 10. Repeat x 3. Turn around and repeat x 3 on the other foot.

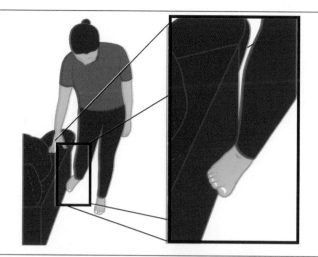

9. Foot Roll In

Stand behind and to the side of a sofa or couch. Stand on the right side of the sofa / couch to exercise the right foot and on the left side of the sofa / couch to exercise the left foot. Hold the back of the sofa / couch to maintain balance. Raise the right foot off the ground and stand only on the left leg. Place the inner aspect of the right foot against the side of the sofa / couch. Now push the right foot inwards and into the sofa / couch. Hold this position for a count of 10. Repeat x 3. Move to the left side of the sofa and repeat x 3 on the left foot.

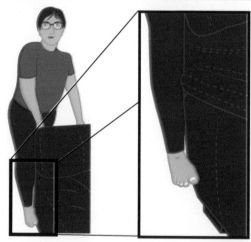

The following four exercises require an exercise resistance band. This is available in most sports stores or can be purchased online. Start with light-coloured bands like yellow and light green, which have less resistance. With time one can progress to tougher bands which are usually black or blue in colour.

10. Band Pull-Out

Hold the ends of the band after looping the band around the right foot. Step on the band with the left foot as shown. Pull on the band to ensure that there is no slack in the band between the left foot and the right foot. Firmly press and hold the band down with the left foot. Now pull and roll out the right foot. Hold this position for a count of 10. Repeat x 3. Swap the band to the opposite side and repeat x 3.

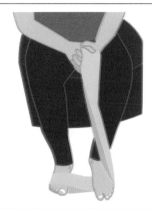

11. Band Pull In

Hold the ends of the band after looping the band around the right foot. Cross legs with the left leg going behind the right. Step on the band with the left foot. Pull-on the band to ensure that there is no slack in the band between the left foot and the right foot. Firmly press and hold the band down with the left foot. Now pull and roll the right foot inwards. Hold it in this position for a count of 10. Repeat x 3. Swap the band to the opposite side and repeat x 3. This exercise can also be done by crossing the leg across the knee as shown in the 2nd and 3rd image.

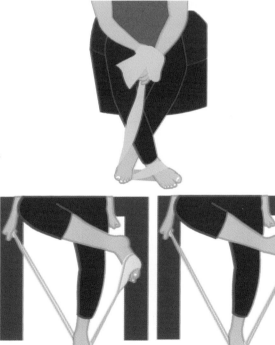

12. Band Pull-Up

Hold the ends of the band after looping the band around the right foot. Step on the band with the left foot and keep the feet together and close to each other. Pull on the band to ensure that there is no slack in the band between the left foot and the right foot. Firmly press and hold the band down with the left foot. Now pull up the right foot. Hold this position for a count of 10. Repeat x 3. Swap the band to the opposite side and repeat x 3.

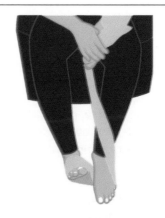

13. Band Push Down

Sit on a chair or couch. Hold the ends of the band after looping the band around the right foot. Loop the middle of the band around the front of the foot. There should not be any slack in the band. Push the foot down. Hold it in this position for a count of 10. Repeat x 3. Swap the band to the opposite side and repeat x 3

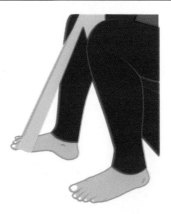

Exercises for Intrinsic muscles

The following seven exercises strengthen the intrinsic muscles of the feet. Two groups of muscles control the foot, called the extrinsic and intrinsic muscles. The larger extrinsic muscles arise from, the lower leg and are responsible for the more significant movements of the foot. The intrinsic muscles are smaller muscles that originate and are located within the foot. They are responsible for the more refined actions of the foot, such as toe control. Some foot conditions create an imbalance between these two groups of muscles, and the extrinsic muscles become much stronger, completely overpowering the intrinsic muscles. This can cause foot pain and deformity. Increasing the strength of the intrinsic muscle is useful to combat this imbalance.

14. Doming

Place feet flat on the floor. Pull the ball (front) of the foot towards the heel. Attempt to increase the arch or dome of the foot. Do not move the toes. If the toes curl up, the exercise is not being done correctly. The intention is to elevate the arch or increase the dome of the foot without curling the toes. Hold for a count of 10. Return to normal. Repeat x 3. The intrinsic muscles help increase the height of the arch (doming) or decrease the length of the foot. If the toes curl, then the extrinsic muscles are being activated, and the exercise is not strengthening the intrinsic muscles as it should. Please note that one can pull back the ball of the feet only by a few millimetres.

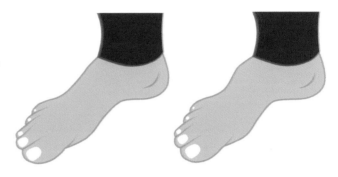

15. Toe Spread Out

Place feet flat on the floor. Spread the toes out as much as possible. Hold this position for a count of 10. Return to normal. Repeat x 3.

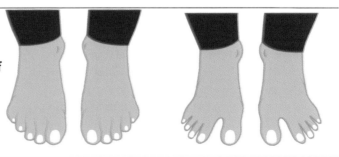

16. Towel Curls

This exercise is best performed on a smooth and polished wooden floor. It is difficult to perform this exercise on a carpeted or tiled floor. Spread a thin towel on the floor. Sit on a chair barefoot and place the feet flat on the floor and the towel. Now repeatedly curl the toes, pulling the towel more and more under the feet with each curl. The towel should scrunch up under the feet. Stop when the end of the towel is reached. Now reverse the process, and push the towel out from under the feet to the front. Spread out the towel once again and repeat the process three times.

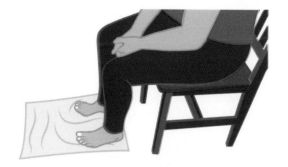

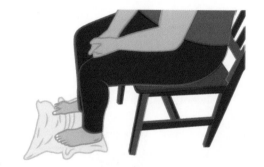

17. Lifting Marbles

Sit on a chair and place five marbles on the floor in front of the right foot. Using the toes of the right foot, grab a marble, lift it, and place it in front of the left foot. Transfer all the 5 marbles to the front of the left foot. Then use the left foot to transfer the marbles back to the front of the right foot. Repeat x 3. Small, crumpled pieces of paper can be used instead of marbles. It has the added advantage of not rolling away.

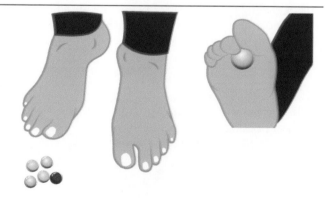

18. Lifting the Toes Up against the Top of the Shoes.

Put shoes on both feet. Once the feet are firmly inside, lift the toes of both feet against the top of the shoes. Hold this position for a count of 10. Repeat x 3.

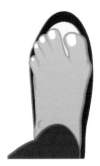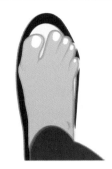

19. Curl the Toes Down Against Soles of Shoes.

Put shoes on both feet. Once the feet are firmly inside, curl the toes of both feet down against the soles of the shoes. Hold this position for a count of 10. Repeat x 3.

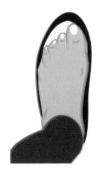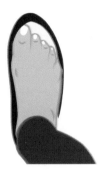

20. Spread the Toes Against the Sides of Shoes

Put shoes on both feet. Once the feet are firmly inside, spread the toes of both feet against the sides of the shoes. Hold this position for a count of 10. Repeat x 3.

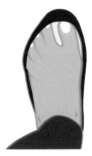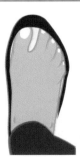

Balance exercises

21. Standing on One Leg

Stand beside a table or a chair. One does not need to hold on to the table or chair; it is just there in case balance is lost. Lift one leg and stand on other leg for a count of 10. Repeat on both legs x 3. One can hold the chair or table if one cannot stand on one leg due to a lack of balance. Slowly as balance improves over the weeks, the hold can be decreased. Progress from holding with both hands, to one hand, to one finger and finally with no hold.

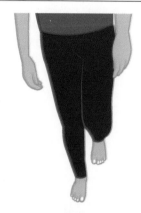

22. Standing On One Leg On a Pillow (do this only after doing 21 comfortably)

Place a pillow on the floor beside a table or a chair. Stand on the pillow with both legs. Slowly raise one leg and stand only on the other leg. Hold onto the table or chair if needed. Gradually as balance improves over the weeks, the hold can be decreased. Progress from holding with both hands, to one hand, to one finger and finally with no hold. Stand for a count of 10. Repeat on the opposite Leg. Repeat on both legs x 3.

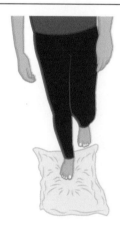

Tap and massage

23. Tap the Floor

While seated comfortably, lift the ball and toes of the feet away from the floor. Then lower the front of the feet and tap them on the floor. Keep the heels resting on the ground at all times. Repeat the process and keep tapping the floor for one whole minute.

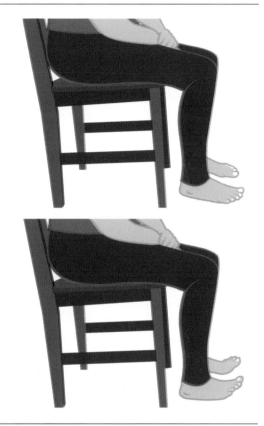

24. Massage with tennis ball

Whilst remaining barefoot, place a tennis ball under the right foot. Apply firm pressure (as tolerated) onto the tennis ball and roll it under the foot. The tennis ball should remain in contact with the sole at all times. Please ensure that the entire sole is used to move the ball. Do this for one minute and then swap to the opposite foot. Repeat x 3.

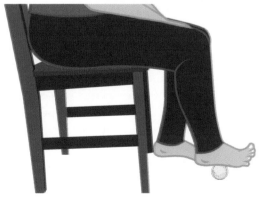

25.   Massage with a fizzy drink can

Whilst remaining barefoot, place a fizzy drink can under the right foot. Apply firm pressure (as tolerated) onto the can and roll it under the foot. The can should remain in contact with the sole at all times. Please ensure that the entire sole is used to move the can. Do this for one minute and then swap to the opposite foot. Repeat x 3. If there is a lot of inflammation, a refrigerated can also be used. Do not use a refrigerated can in case of diabetes or neuropathy (numbness in the feet).

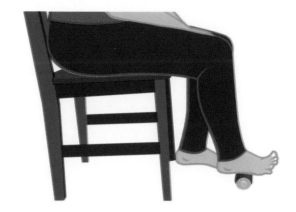

References

1. Gates LS, Arden NK, Hannan MT, Roddy E, Gill TK, Hill CL, Dufour AB, Rathod-Mistry T, Thomas MJ, Menz HB, Bowen CJ, Golightly YM. Prevalence of Foot Pain Across an International Consortium of Population-Based Cohorts. Arthritis Care Res (Hoboken). 2019 May;71(5):661-670.

2. Macera A, Carulli C, Sirleo L, Innocenti M. Postoperative Complications and Reoperation Rates Following Open Reduction and Internal Fixation of Ankle Fracture. Joints. 2018 May 21;6(2):110-115.

3. Barg A, Harmer JR, Presson AP, Zhang C, Lackey M, Saltzman CL. Unfavorable Outcomes Following Surgical Treatment of Hallux Valgus Deformity: A Systematic Literature Review. J Bone Joint Surg Am. 2018 Sep 19;100(18):1563-1573.

4. Rewhorn MJ, Leung AH, Gillespie A, Moir JS, Miller R. Incidence of complex regional pain syndrome after foot and ankle surgery. J Foot Ankle Surg. 2014 May-Jun;53(3):256-8.

5. Lewis RD, Wright P, McCarthy LH. Orthotics Compared to Conventional Therapy and Other Non-Surgical Treatments for Plantar Fasciitis. J Okla State Med Assoc. 2015 Dec;108(12):596-8.

6. Männikkö K, Sahlman J. The Effect of Metatarsal Padding on Pain and Functional Ability in Metatarsalgia. Scand J Surg. 2017 Dec;106(4):332-337.

7. Aebischer AS, Duff S. Bunions: A review of management. Aust J Gen Pract. 2020 Nov;49(11):720-723.

8. Farzadi M, Safaeepour Z, Mousavi ME, Saeedi H. Effect of medial arch support foot orthosis on plantar pressure distribution in females with mild-to-moderate hallux valgus after one month of follow-up. Prosthet Orthot Int. 2015 Apr;39(2):134-9.

9. van Netten JJ, Lazzarini PA, Armstrong DG, et al. Diabetic Foot Australia guideline on footwear for people with diabetes. J Foot Ankle Res. 2018;11:2.

10. Chen TH, Chou LW, Tsai MW, Lo MJ, Kao MJ. Effectiveness of a heel cup with an arch support insole on the standing balance of the elderly. Clin Interv Aging. 2014 Feb 20;9:351-6. doi: 10.2147/CIA.S56268.

11. Landorf KB, Ackland CA, Bonanno DR, Menz HB, Forghany S. Effects of metatarsal domes on plantar pressures in older people with a history of forefoot pain. J Foot Ankle Res. 2020 May 6;13(1):18.

12. Halstead J, Chapman GJ, Gray JC, Grainger AJ, Brown S, Wilkins RA, Roddy E, Helliwell PS, Keenan AM, Redmond AC. Foot orthoses in the treatment of symptomatic midfoot osteoarthritis using clinical and biomechanical outcomes: a randomised feasibility study. Clin Rheumatol. 2016 Apr;35(4):987-96..

13. Bonanno DR, Murley GS, Munteanu SE, Landorf KB, Menz HB. Foot orthoses for the prevention of lower limb overuse injuries in naval recruits: study protocol for a randomised controlled trial. J Foot Ankle Res. 2015 Sep 11;8:51.

14. Arnold MJ, Moody AL. Common Running Injuries: Evaluation and Management. Am Fam Physician. 2018 Apr 15;97(8):510-516.

15. Van Alsenoy K, Ryu JH, Girard O. The Effect of EVA and TPU Custom Foot Orthoses on Running Economy, Running Mechanics, and Comfort. Front Sports Act Living. 2019 Sep 19;1:34.

Printed in Great Britain
by Amazon

24686711R00027